Med

Beginners

How To Relieve Stress, Anxiety And Depression, Find Inner Peace And Happiness

Introduction

I want to thank you and congratulate you for downloading the book, *"Meditation For Beginners - How To Relieve Stress, Anxiety And Depression, Find Inner Peace And Happiness."* This book contains proven steps and strategies on how to meditate effectively to enjoy the benefits meditation has to offer.

Experts have rightly described meditation as the 'art of living' owing to its ability to help you disengage from the autopilot mode, discover your true self, live a more loving and caring life, be present at all times, find the capacity to live your life more wisely, and deal with mental conditions such as depression, stress, and anxiety.

Millions of people meditate for different reasons such as religion and therapy just to mention a few. Whether you choose to meditate for religious or therapeutic reasons, the truth remains that meditation can help change the way you generally approach life, the way you react to life's circumstances, and how you relate and interact with the people in your life.

In this meditation guide for beginners, we shall discuss and understand everything you need to know about meditation before you start practicing it and how best to meditate to reap the amazing benefits meditation has to offer.

Thanks again for downloading this book, I hope you enjoy it!

Table of Contents

Meditation: Why You Should Make It A Daily Habit

We live in a world where things do not always work out as planned. As such, we have to change our plans to match our constantly changing situations. If you look back a few years, you will discover a number of goals and dreams you could not accomplish despite all your efforts.

When things keep going wrong and the future appears not to hold a lot of promise, depression, stress, and anxiety can easily set in. Unfortunately, when it comes to managing these conditions, medical treatments may not be as effective, which necessitates the mastery of a natural technique that can help you deal with these conditions and live a happier life. Meditation is that technique: meditation helps your mind gain more mental clarity, concentration, stability, calmness, emotional positivity, and helps you see things as they really are. But what exactly is meditation?

Understanding Meditation

Meditation has come a long way and over the years, witnessed a number of modifications to suit specific goals. Most individuals see meditation as an exercise that helps them slow down and eventually succeed at stopping the ceaseless flow of random thoughts.

While this is indeed true, it does not really explain what meditation is despite capturing the essence of meditation. Simply put, we can define meditation as a *state of thoughtless awareness.*

Meditation is not about what you do, it is all about being aware of what you do, how you do it, how long you do it, and how doing it makes you feel. You can sit in the lotus yoga posture in a very serene garden and still be very far from meditating while someone else can go about his daily chores while meditating by maintaining mindful awareness of every single step he/she takes, the sights, sounds and sensations associated with the particular chores or activities he/she engages in.

Now that you understand what meditation is, you may be wondering, how does meditation work? To help you understand this, we need to look at how meditation affects you especially how it affects your brain. Let us do that now!

How Meditation Affects Your Brain

Most books write about meditation and its effectiveness at treating mental issues such as depression, anxiety, stress, etc., without first trying to discuss why this seemingly simple mental exercise is an effective remedy against these conditions.

This book is not like the many others out there and as such, before we discuss how meditation benefits you, it is important we discuss how meditation affects you. Fortunately, scores of research studies point to the correlation between meditation and the health of your brain, which explains its effectiveness at treating and managing the previously mentioned conditions.

According to reports from results of research conducted by Sarah Lazar and her team at Harvard University, mindful meditation changes the structure of the human brain. The results from their study showed that meditation increases the cortical thickness of the hippocampus, the part of the brain responsible for memory and learning.

The research study also recorded a drastic reduction in the volume of brain cells in the amygdala, the part of the brain responsible for regulating anxiety, stress, and fear. The change in the volume of the brain cells in the amygdala explained why participants recorded visible reduction in stress and anxiety levels.

In another study conducted by Dr. Alderman and his team of researchers at Rutgers University, N.J., results of MRI scans of the brains of people who engaged in meditation for about 8 weeks showed increased amount of gray matter in the prefrontal cortex, the area of the brain responsible for controlling attention and focus.

The increase of gray matter in the prefrontal cortex is responsible for reduced rumination over unpleasant past events that have hitherto kept the participants depressed.

The effects meditation has on your brain may not be enough to make meditation effective at treating anxiety, depression, stress, or whatever mental condition you are trying to overcome until you make this mindful exercise a daily habit. In a later section, this book will show you how to make meditation a daily habit.

For now, let us continue our discussion by discussing how meditation benefits you.

How Meditation Benefits You

Meditation can make your life better in several ways. In fact, the benefits of meditation are as numerous as they are far-reaching. Once you learn to live in the moment, you can concentrate on living a great life, concentrate on things that matter the most, and pay attention to vital details at hand rather than brooding over your past mistakes and future worries.

Here are the various ways meditation benefits you

1: Sustains Your Brain's Ability to Recall

It is natural for the human brain to lose its cognitive ability as you age; however, studies by researchers at Harvard University have shown that because of the proliferation of gray matter in certain vital parts of your brain such as the hippocampus, engaging in mindful meditation can help your brain's memorizing ability.

2: Prevents High Blood Pressure

According to results of researches on the effects of meditation on high blood pressure as published in the Journal of Alternative and Complementary Medicine, meditating regularly helps you relax by increasing the Nitric Oxide content in your blood.

Nitric Oxide is responsible for the opening of the blood vessels, and consequently, a drop in blood pressure. According to the report, those who meditated regularly stopped taking their drugs a couple of weeks after engaging in the practice.

3: Helps You Beat Depression, Stress and Anxiety

We often spend most of our time worrying about what tomorrow may bring and regretting certain decisions and choices we made in the past. As we age, these worries and regrets build up stress, anxiety, and depression.

Engaging in mindful meditation helps you clear your thoughts of all such worries, fears, regrets, and helps you concentrate on the present and enjoy life moment-to-moment.

4: Helps You Maintain Peace of Mind and Happiness

Dedicating a couple of minutes every day to meditate is a sure way to stay in the right mood, maintain high energy level, enjoy peace of mind, stay happy by appreciating the beautiful and free gifts of nature that you often ignore, etc.

When you form the habit of meditating daily, you become more aware of your environment, and the more aware you become, the more you tend to take note of seemingly insignificant things that could brighten your day.

For instance, by engaging in meditation, you start noticing things such as the rustling of leaves in the backyard, the chirping of birds in the bush, the sound of raindrops as they hit your roof, the sensation of warm water caressing your skin, the sound of a baby giggling, etc.

5: Improves Your Self-Discipline

Meditation helps you become more attentive to things that matter in your life. When you start meditating, you will start taking note of how you spend your time and how much time you spend on a particular task. Meditation will also help you take note of the activities that bring out the best of your moods and the tasks that drain your energy and happiness. Once you become aware of how much time you spend on tasks, and how this makes you feel, you will be in a position to decide if such a task or activity is worth your time and effort. This is why most self-development experts' advice their clients to engage in meditation as a way of overcoming a particular bad habit. Suffice it to say, meditation helps you build character and good habits that all boil down to self-discipline.

6: Improves Your Overall Health Condition

According to Herbert Benson, a Harvard University Medical School researcher, meditation, and relaxation go hand-in-hand in that relaxation is either the goal of a meditation exercise or the result of it.

Based on his studies and his results, meditation leads to the reduction of several health conditions. The main benefit of meditation is in respect to the activities and state of the nervous system. According to the research, some of the health benefits of meditation include:

* *Improved blood circulation*
* *Reduced palpitation*
* *Reduced perspiration*
* *Slower rate of respiration*
* *Reduced anxiety*
* *Greater feelings of wellbeing*

Reduced stress levels
Deeper relaxation
Lower level of blood cortisol, etc.

Most of the benefits of meditation mentioned above are possible because meditation affects the parts of your brain that regulate psychological conditions such as mood, anxiety, worry, depression, stress, etc.

Now that we have that out of the way, let us now look at the general guidelines you need to know as you seek to engage in effective meditation that helps you derive all the stated benefits:

General Guidelines For Effective Meditation

As you start creating room for meditation in your life, here are the various things you need to know to make your practice and meditation session as effective is possible:

1: You Need the Most Conducive Environment

Inasmuch as you can easily sit anywhere and anyhow to meditate, you should consider the quietness and privacy of the location you have chosen as your meditation zone.

The need for quietness and privacy during meditation links to the fact that the less interruption you experience as you meditate, the more likely you are to get the best results from your meditation.

As such, find a very secluded and serene spot in your home, school, or office and designate it as your meditation spot. The moment you have a place you can always use when you want to engage in mindful meditation, it becomes easier to concentrate and achieve complete mindfulness during your meditation session.

-Round Cotton Zafu Meditation Cushion-

2: Have a Specific Time for Meditation

No one is saying you cannot choose to meditate at random and on impulse. The point here is that you should have a specific time in your daily routine timetable allocated to mindful meditation. This time can be at any time of the day depending on the nature of your job and all other activities you do during the day.

To achieve maximum results, choose between the early hours of the morning before you embark on your daily chores or the hours before bedtime. You do not have to meditate for one whole hour especially if you are just beginning; wanting to do this may make the whole exercise appear difficult or even impossible.

As a beginner, limit the duration of your meditation sessions to about 5 minutes, but of course with time, you can always increase the duration as your brain and body accustoms to meditation.

3: Pay Attention to Your Breath

The best way to focus on your breath is to make sure you breathe in slowly and deeply. First, start by lowering your unfocused gaze towards your stomach. Breathe in slowly without trying to force your breaths, let your breaths come naturally as you breathe in through your nose and out through your mouth.

At first, the breaths will come in shallow gasps that will not last long, but with time, your airways will get fuller with air and your breaths are bound to last longer as you breathe in and out. Do not try to manipulate the duration of each breath; simply let the air go in and out of your airways at its own pace.

4: Be Mindful

As your breath becomes fuller and deeper, you will naturally notice that your nerves and muscles will begin to feel calmer. Notice the rise and fall of your stomach as the air makes its way through your nostrils and out of your mouth. To enhance the effects of your mindful awareness, take note of the time it takes for each breath to go in and the time it takes to come out. No matter how full or deep each breath is, it cannot last more than a couple of seconds. You can simply take note of the duration by counting the number of seconds it takes you to breathe in and the number of seconds it takes you to breathe out using your fingers or simply taking note of it in your mind.

Occasionally, you will notice your mind straying from being attentive to your breaths. Whenever this happens, which will probably be a number of times, do not lose focus; your ability to take note of what just happened is a good indication that you are in a state of awareness. As you develop your power of focus, it will become easier to concentrate and pay attention.

5: Ending Each Meditation Session

When it comes to ending your meditation, you should not just get up, fold up your mat if you have any, and walk away. It is important that you remain mindful and conscious of your state of awareness even as you end each meditation session. When you are ready to end your meditation session, you should begin by gently opening your eyes, and get up slowly. Engage in some light stretching and make sure you transfer your state of awareness to the very act of stretching your body by noticing if you feel pains in any of the joints or if you hear any sounds as the joints straighten.

Even after stretching, you should transfer thoughtful awareness to the next activity you engage in such as walking back to your home if you had gone to the garden, porch, or backyard to observe the mindful meditation.

Following the guidelines outlined here will ensure you get the best from your meditation sessions. However, how do you ensure that you don't just meditate for a week and not bother about meditation again. Let us learn how to make meditation a habit in the following chapter.

How To Make Meditation A Habit

When it comes to building any new habit you consider important enough to incorporate into your daily life, you need motivation and several other factors that can help you start and stay strong until you succeed.
Below is a simple step-by-step guide you can use to make meditation a part of your daily life to beat stress, depression, fear, anxiety, and live a happier life.

1: Identify Your Core Values

What are values? The first thing you must understand is that your values are dissimilar to someone else's. Your values are the things you think about, talk about, read about, and learn about every day. If you do not know your values or you think you have no values, here is a set of questions that can help you discover your core values:
* Apart from work, how do you spend most of your time at work?
* Whenever you get your monthly paycheck or any financial incentive, what is the first thing you spend the money on?
* What type of things do you enjoy researching and learning about more than other things?
* What area of your life do you feel you are best at?
* What is your greatest inspiration in life?
If someone asked you to choose one thing you would love to achieve in the next ten years, what would that be?
* What do you find yourself dreaming about and desiring most of the time?

2: Consider How Meditation Will Affect Your Core Values

Now that you have defined your core values from the answers you got from the above exercise, you know the things you term most important. The next step is to find a way to link your core values to the meditation exercise you want to master.

Let us take for instance; your values are rooted in any of the following areas of your life: parenting, profession, spirituality, or creativity. Here are some possible effects meditation will have on your core values.

Parenting
Meditation will help you stay calm enough not to snap at your kids
Meditation can help you build your character and become a good role model for your kids
Meditation helps you understand your child through awareness and fosters a deeper connection with them.
When things go wrong, and everyone seems to get on your nerves, meditation helps you stay calm.

Profession
Meditation will help you make informed business and organizational decisions.
Meditation will give you the concentration you need to focus on your job responsibilities and improve productivity.
Meditation makes you a better listener, a vital component of effective communication. Effective communication is a leadership quality you need in truckloads.
Meditation will help you deal with conflicts at the workplace.
Meditation will enable you replenish lost energy after the day's work stress.

Creativity
Meditation will help you understand your emotions better and productively channel them.
Meditation will enhance your creativity.
Meditation makes you more focused and better at what you do.

Meditation will help you generate beautiful ideas you can then translate into things like poetry, paintings, drawings, songs, books, etc.
Meditation will make you appreciate art better as you begin to view art in new light or appreciation.
Meditation helps you connect to a higher power from where you can get inspiration.

Spirituality
Meditation will give you deeper insight into spiritual things.
Meditation will keep your self-awareness straightened, which acts as the base of every spiritual transformation and virtue.
Meditation gives you better control over your instincts and emotions, thus helping you live a more spiritually inclined life.
Meditation frees you from every negativity and mental bondage.
Meditation helps you live your life as creation intended it for you.
Why is identification of core values and the possibly effects of meditation on them important? The answer is simple: *the moment you identify your core values in life and establish how meditation helps you keep them alive, it becomes easier to commit to regular meditation and make it a daily habit.*

3: Pen Everything Down On Paper

Write down the core values you identified as the values that matter the most to you and make a list of at least five ways meditation helps you sustain each of the core values you have listed. Place the paper where you can easily spot it several times a day so it can serve as a reminder and a motivator to stick to your daily meditation plans.

4: Make a Clear Commitment to Daily Meditation

Do not simply say, "I will make sure I spend some minutes every morning meditating." This will not motivate you enough to get you started. Instead, have something clearer, more detailed, and specific such as, "I will meditate for five minutes in my study and on my yoga mat at 5:30" Notice the elements mentioned in this statement:

Time: Every 5:30 am
Duration: 5 minutes
Location: Study
Tool: Yoga mat; your tools can also include your alarm clock or a stopwatch to help you keep to time.

When you have such a clear and specific schedule for your daily meditation, a schedule that considers these four important elements, it should take less than two weeks before you start looking forward to each meditation session.

5: Design Some Triggers

Because of one reason or the other, it is actually easy to forget or skip your meditation session. To ensure this does not happen, you have to find a way to design some reminders. Here are some common examples:

Set an alarm: Undoubtedly, your phone should have an alarm device or you can get a small alarm clock and place it on a small table beside your bed.

You can set the alarm to sound 10 minutes before the time you wake up (if you have chosen the morning time). If you have chosen any other time of the day to meditate, you can set a reminder on your phone 10 minutes to the time, you have allocated to meditation.

The reminder message can read something like, "Your meditation starts in 10 minutes." This will help you disengage from whatever you were doing in that particular moment, and give your meditation the attention it deserves.

* *Paste a reminder on the mirror in your bathroom:* Most people look in the mirror to see how they look each morning – we all impulsively do this. Pasting a paper reading, "*Do not forget your morning meditation to get rid of stress, depression, anxiety*, will help you swing into action.

6: Be Accountable To Someone

It helps to share your meditation plans and goals with someone or some people before you begin. You can announce your decision to start meditating and the reason for the meditation on your Facebook, Twitter, or other social media platforms.

You can also confide in your spouse, a friend, or family member about your decision to meditate. This will help you stick to the new habit because you know you have to report your progress to someone as you progress.

7: Learn More about Meditation

You can download some meditation videos online, watch some meditation sessions on YouTube, seek new friends who meditate, read books on meditation, join meditation forums online, etc. All these will help build up your knowledge, clarity, expertise, and commitment to meditation.

8: Cultivate the 'No Matter What Attitude'

Occasionally, you will find yourself in situations that may easily discourage you from meditating. However, when you make up your mind that you must meditate for at least 5 minutes every morning, you will find your way around every obstacle.

For instance, if you find yourself in a situation that requires you to leave home before the time you have allocated to meditation, you will wake up a bit earlier to accommodate your meditation session before leaving home.

Once you make meditation a habit, it becomes easier to use meditation to treat any mental condition. The next section talks about how you can use meditation to overcome depression.

How To Meditate To Overcome Depression

As you may already know, an inability to stop unhappy memories and gloomy thoughts from the past from ceaselessly invading your mind characterizes depression. According to researchers, this pattern of thinking called rumination, affects two distinct parts of the brain: the prefrontal cortex, and the hippocampus.

The prefrontal cortex controls focus and attention, while the hippocampus controls learning and memory. According to Dr. Brandon Alderman from Rutgers University in New Jersey, depressed people have a much smaller hippocampus than people who are not dealing with depression.

According to Alderman, brain scan studies have shown that people who meditate experience better brain-cell communications in the prefrontal cortex when taking cognitive tests than people who do not meditate.

This increase in brain-cell communication at the prefrontal cortex, as most researchers believe, is the reason why people who engage in meditation can concentrate and focus on the present better than those who do not. This easily explains why meditation can help you stay focused, entertain less depressive thoughts, and eliminate depression.

The same research studies by researchers at Rutgers University have shown that meditation helps depressed people snap out of their depression by becoming more aware of the present and forgetting their unpleasant pasts.

One other effective way meditation can help you get rid of depression is by stimulating the release of the feel good hormone such as serotonin.

There are a number of very simple meditation steps you can use to overcome your depressive state. Here are some of these steps:

1. Get a seat that allows you to sit with your back straightened. Sit straight and place your feet on the floor.

2. Shut your eyes and utilize all your imaginative power to imagine the flow of air in and out of your respiratory system. Be mindful of every sensation, and avoid passing judgment on the experience. You do not have to manipulate your breathing; just let it flow naturally and calmly.

3. It is normal for your mind to wander off after sometime. Initially, this will happen often, but with time, it should become less frequent. Whenever you catch your mind wandering off, simply stop the confused flow of thoughts, and refocus your thoughts on your breath.

Do not worry if your thoughts wander off for a long time without your notice. The art of mastering your thoughts is a gradual process that takes time to master.

4. After practicing this mindful meditation for about 5-10 minutes, you will notice a natural calmness settling in your mind. Repeating this technique at least once a day for a couple of weeks should give you full control over your thoughts and help you get rid of every trace of anxiety.

Depression is not the only mental condition meditation can help you manage and eliminate. You can also use meditation to remove stress from your life. The next section focuses on the meditation technique you should adopt to reduce your stress levels.

Using Meditation For Stress Relief

Researchers at Stanford carried out an 8-week study on mindfulness. Their intention was to ascertain meditation's effectiveness at reducing stress. From the results of the study, they found that the rate of activity in the prefrontal cortex, the part of the brain responsible for regulating emotions increased.

The increased activity in the prefrontal cortex led to the reduction of stress levels. Similarly, researchers at Harvard University discovered specific changes in the structure of the brain following meditation. The change in brain structure showed meditation's ability to regulate emotions that can lead to stress.

One major meditation technique that can help you manage stress easily is mindful deep breathing. Researchers have linked meditation's ability to help you deal with stress to the reduction of cortisol produced by your adrenal gland. Cortisol is your body's main stress hormone; any reduction in its production means less stress for you.

Cortisol production begins when the amygdala sends specific signals about an impending threat to the hippocampus. The hippocampus in turn signals the adrenal gland to produce cortisol. When you practice deep breathing, the rate of activity in the amygdala part of your brain reduces, and the rate at which the amygdala sends signals to your hippocampus reduces.

This reduction in activities in the amygdala and the rate at which information reaches the hippocampus from the amygdala means your body produces a much smaller amount of cortisol. The more you practice deep breathing, the more this chain repeats, and the less stressed you feel.

Deep Breathing Meditation Technique

The major difference between deep breathing and normal breathing is that in deep breathing, you draw air from your abdomen to ensure you fill up your lungs with each drawn breath. Drawing deeply from your abdomen ensures you never run short of breath, feel tense, or anxious.

Below are some steps you can take to achieve the best results:

1. Get comfortably seated with your back straight. Place one hand on your abdomen.

2. Deeply draw in air through your nostrils and take note of the rise and fall of the hand placed on your abdomen with each breath you take.

3. Exhale through your mouth and as you do, release as much air as you can, and allow the muscles at your abdomen to contract. Take note of the movement of the hand on your abdomen as you exhale.

4. Continue inhaling through your nostrils and exhaling through your mouth. Drawing in enough air will make the rising and falling movement of your abdomen more obvious. To become more aware, you can count the number of seconds it takes to exhale each time.

5. For a more calming effect that helps you feel less stressed and calmer, as you practice deep breathing meditation, listen to soulful music.

Just as meditation helps you deal with depression and stress, you can also use it to eliminate anxiety. Here is how:

Using Meditation To Ease Anxiety

Anxiety is the other mental condition meditation can help you effectively deal with.

Whether you are a born worrier or your worry emanates from the many stressful situations you have to deal with, you constantly experience racing thoughts that refuse to go away. This is where meditation comes in.

Meditation can help quiet your over active mind. Meditation helps you detach from thoughts and feelings that make you anxious. In fact, meditation is all about remaining grounded and centered.

Constant meditation helps you learn how to return to your grounded state. However and as stated earlier, to derive the benefits of meditation, you have to make it a daily habit. Below is a simple technique you can use to live a less anxious life:

1. Find a calm place where you can relax and put your thoughts in order. If you choose a noisy place for meditation, you may not get the long-term results you desire.

2. Choose a convenient time for your daily meditations to beat your anxiety. If you do not have a specific time dedicated to meditation, it may not be easy to make meditation a daily habit.

3. Experiment with different positions such as sitting, standing, or lying positions to help you choose the most appropriate and comfortable position for your meditation exercise.

4. The moment you choose a particular place, time, and sitting position, the best way to begin your meditation is to concentrate on the flow of air in and out of your airways.

5. Practice deep breathing and concentrate on how air rushes down your air pipe and the sound it makes while going and coming out.

6. Count the number of seconds it takes you to complete each breath; you can also count the number of breaths you take per minute.

7. Pay attention to your breath and nothing else. If you notice your thoughts drifting from your breath to an event, place, person, or whatever keeps you worried and anxious, simply refocus your attention on your breath.

8. Develop a mantra to direct your thoughts towards; you can choose words or even phrases that evoke feelings of peace and calmness. Some examples of mantras you can choose include "Walking in a beautiful garden," "sound of raindrops," "singing angels," etc. Anything that can give you a feeling of peace and tranquility will do.

9. For a start, dedicate about 5-10 minutes every day and increase the duration when you have mastered the act of meditation.

10. Just as you began mindfully, do not forget to end your meditation in a mindful way that helps you transfer the awareness to every other thing you involve yourself in all through the day.

Conclusion

Thank you again for downloading this book!
I hope this book was able to help you to learn about meditation.
The next step is to start meditating today and reap the many benefits meditation has to offer.

Finally, if you enjoyed this book, you be kind enough to leave a review for this book on Amazon?

Click here to leave a book review on Amazon!
Thank you and good luck!

Printed in Great Britain
by Amazon